Sushma Rakasi

Pinaverium sustained release matrix tablets for colonic drug delivery

Sajal Kumar Jha
Sushma Rakasi

Pinaverium sustained release matrix tablets for colonic drug delivery

LAP LAMBERT Academic Publishing

Imprint

Any brand names and product names mentioned in this book are subject to trademark, brand or patent protection and are trademarks or registered trademarks of their respective holders. The use of brand names, product names, common names, trade names, product descriptions etc. even without a particular marking in this work is in no way to be construed to mean that such names may be regarded as unrestricted in respect of trademark and brand protection legislation and could thus be used by anyone.

Cover image: www.ingimage.com

Publisher:
LAP LAMBERT Academic Publishing
is a trademark of
International Book Market Service Ltd., member of OmniScriptum Publishing Group
17 Meldrum Street, Beau Bassin 71504, Mauritius

ISBN: 978-620-2-55458-9

TABLE OF CONTENTS

ABSTRACT

In the present work sustained release matrix formulation of Pinaverium targeted to colon by using various polymers is developed. To facilitate the pH-independent drug release of Pinaverium, pH modifying agents (buffering agents) were used. Colon targeted tablets were prepared in two steps. Initially core tablets were prepared then the tablets were coated with Ph dependent polymers. Eudragit RLPO and S100 were used as enteric coating polymers. The pre-compression mixture of all formulations was subjected to various flow property tests and each one the formulations were passed the tests. The tablets were coated by polymers and so the coated tablets were subjected to various evaluation techniques. The tablets were passed all the tests. Among all the formulations F6 formulation was found to be optimized as a result of it had the drug release of up to 12 hours and showed most of 98.45% drug release. It followed zero- order mechanism.

Keywords: Pinaverium, Colon targeted drug delivery system, ethyl group polysaccharide, Eudragit RLPO, Eudragit S 100

2

INTRODUCTION:

Targeted drug delivery into the colon is extremely fascinating for native treatment of a range of viscous diseases like inflammatory bowel disease, Crohn's sickness, amoebiasis, colonic cancer, native treatment of colonic pathologies, and general delivery of super molecule and amide medicine.1,2 The colon is believed to be an appropriate absorption website for peptides and super molecule medicine for the subsequent reasons; (i) less diversity, and intensity of organic process enzymes, (ii) comparative chemical action activity of colon tissue layer is way but that discovered within the bowel, therefore CDDS protects amide medicine from chemical reaction, and catalyst degradation in small intestine and small intestine, and eventually releases the drug into small intestine or colon that ends up in larger general bioavailability.4 and eventually, as a result of the colon encompasses a long duration that is up to five days and is extremely attentive to absorption enhancers.5

Oral route is that the most convenient and most well-liked route however different routes for CDDS could also be used. body part administration offers the shortest route for targeting medicine to the colon. However, reaching the proximal a part of colon via body part administration is tough. Body part administration also can be uncomfortable for patients and compliance could also be but optimum.6 Drug preparation for intrarectal administration is provided as solutions, foam, and suppositories. The intrarectal route is employed each as a method of general dosing and for the delivery of locally active drug to the massive internal organ. Corticosteroids like Hydrocortone and anti-inflammatory ar administered via the body part for the treatment of inflammatory bowel disease. though these medicine are absorbed from the massive viscous, it's typically believed that their effectiveness is due principally to the topical application. The concentration of drug reaching the colon depends on formulation factors, the extent of retrograde spreading and therefore the retention time. Foam and suppositories are shown to be maintained principally within the body part and colon whereas irrigation solutions have an excellent spreading capability.7

Because of the high water absorption capability of the colon, the colonic contents are significantly viscous and their intermixture isn't economical, therefore accessibility of most medicine to the assimilative membrane is low. The human colon has over four hundred distinct species of microorganism as resident flora, a potential

3

population of upto 1010 microorganism per gram of colonic contents. Among the reactions disbursed by these gut flora are azoreduction and catalyst cleavage i.e. glycosides.8 These metabolic processes even be|is also} to blame for the metabolism of the many medicine and will also be applied to colon-targeted delivery of amide based mostly macromolecules like hormone by oral administration.

Target sites, colonic disease conditions, and drugs used for treatment are shown in Table 1.9

Table 1

Colon targeting diseases, drugs and sites

Target sites	Disease conditions	Drug and active agents
Topical action	Inflammatory Bowel Diseases, Irritable bowel disease and Crohn's disease. Chronic pancreatitis	Hydrocortisone, Budenoside, Prednisolone, Sulfaselazine, Olsalazine, Mesalazine, Balsalazide.
Local action	Pancreatactomy and cystic fibrosis, Colorectal cancer	Digestive enzyme supplements 5-Flourouracil.
Systemic action	To prevent gastric irritation To prevent first pass metabolism of orally ingested drugs Oral delivery of peptides Oral delivery of vaccines	NSAIDS Steroids Insulin Typhoid

Advantages of CDDS over Conventional Drug Delivery:

Chronic colitis, namely ulcerative colitis, and Crohn's disease are currently treated with glucocorticoids, and other anti-inflammatory agents.[10] Administration of glucocorticoids namely dexamethasone and methyl prednisolone by oral and intravenous routes produce systemic side effects including adenosuppression, immunosuppression, cushinoid symptoms, and bone resorption.[11]

Criteria for Selection of Drug for CDDS:

The best Candidates for CDDS are drugs which show poor absorption from the stomach or intestine including peptides. The drugs used in the treatment of IBD, ulcerative colitis, diarrhea, and colon cancer are ideal candidates for local colon delivery.[13] The criteria for selection of drugs for CDDS is summarized in Table 2.[14-16]

Table 2:

Criteria for selection of drugs for CDDS

Criteria	Pharmacological class	Non-peptide drugs	Peptide drugs
Drugs used for local effects in colon against GIT diseases	Anti-inflammatory drugs	Oxyprenolol, Metoprolol, Nifedipine	Amylin, Antisense oligonucleotide
Drugs poorly absorbed from upper GIT	Antihypertensive and antianginal drugs	Ibuprofen, Isosorbides, Theophylline	Cyclosporine, Desmopressin
Drugs for colon cancer	Antineoplastic drugs	Pseudoephedrine	Epoetin, Glucagon
Drugs that degrade in stomach and small intestine	Peptides and proteins	Bromophenaramine, 5-Flourouracil, Doxorubicin	Gonadoreline, Insulin, Interferons

Criteria	Pharmacological class	Non-peptide drugs	Peptide drugs
Drugs that undergo extensive first pass metabolism	Nitroglycerin and corticosteroids	Bleomycin, Nicotine	Protirelin,sermorelin, Saloatonin
Drugs for targeting	Antiarthritic and antiasthamatic drugs	Prednisolone, hydrocortisone, 5-Amino-salicylic acid	Somatropin,Urotoilitin

Drug Carrier is another factor which influences CDDS. The selection of carrier for particular drugs depends on the physiochemical nature of the drug as well as the disease for which the system is to be used. Factors such as chemical nature, stability and partition coefficient of the drug and type of absorption enhancer chosen influence the carrier selection. Moreover, the choice of drug carrier depends on the functional groups of the drug molecule.[17] For example, aniline or nitro groups on a drug may be used to link it to another benzene group through an azo bond. The carriers, which contain additives like polymers (may be used as matrices and hydro gels or coating agents) may influence the release properties and efficacy of the systems.[13]

Approaches used for Site Specific Drug Delivery to Colon (CDDS)

Several approaches are used for site-specific drug delivery. Among the primary approaches for CDDS, These include:

1) Primary Approaches for CDDS

a. pH Sensitive Polymer Coated Drug Delivery to the Colon:

In the abdomen, hydrogen ion concentration ranges between one and a pair of throughout abstinence however will increase when intake.[18] The hydrogen ion concentration is regarding half dozen.5 within the proximal intestine, and regarding seven.5 within the distal intestine.[19] From the small intestine to the colon, hydrogen ion concentration declines considerably. it's regarding half dozen.4 within the caecum. However, hydrogen ion concentration values as low as five.7 are measured within the colon in healthy volunteers.20 The hydrogen ion concentration within the colon is half dozen.6 and 7.0 within the colon. Use of hydrogen ion concentration dependent polymers relies on these variations in hydrogen ion concentration levels. The polymers delineate as hydrogen ion concentration dependent in colon specific drug delivery ar insoluble at low hydrogen ion concentration levels however become more and more soluble as hydrogen ion concentration rises.21 though a hydrogen ion concentration dependent chemical compound will shield a formulation within the abdomen, and proximal intestine, it's going to begin to dissolve within the lower intestine, and therefore the site-specificity of formulations is poor.22 The decline in hydrogen ion concentration from the tip of the tiny viscus to the colon can even lead to issues, extended lag times at the ileo-cecal junction or mass rapid transit through the colon which may conjointly lead to poor site-specificity of enteric-coated single-unit formulations.21

b. Delayed (Time Controlled Release System) Release Drug Delivery to Colon:

Time controlled unleash system (TCRS) like sustained or delayed unleash dose forms are terribly promising drug unleash systems. However, because of probably giant variations of stomachal removal time of dose forms in humans, in these approaches, colon point in time of dose forms can not be accurately expected, leading to poor colonical accessibility.23 The dose forms may be applicable as colon targeting dose forms by prolonging the lag time of concerning five to six h. However, the disadvantages of this method are:

i.   Stomachal removal time varies markedly between subjects or in a very manner passionate about kind and quantity of food intake.

ii.   GI movement, particularly body process or contraction within the abdomen would end in amendment in gi transit of the drug.24

iii.   Accelerated transit through totally different regions of the colon has been ascertained in patients with the IBD, the tumour syndrome and symptom, and also the colitis.9,25,26

7

Therefore, time dependent systems don't seem to be ideal to deliver medicine to the colon specifically for the treatment of colon connected diseases. applicable integration of pH scale sensitive and time unleash functions into one dose kind could improve the positioning specificity of drug delivery to the colon. Since the transit time of dose forms within the bowel is a smaller amount variable i.e. concerning 3 ± 1 unit of time.27 The time-release perform (or timer function) ought to work additional with efficiency within the bowel as compared the abdomen. within the bowel drug carrier are delivered to the target facet, and drug unleash can begin at a planned time conversion stomachal removal. On the opposite hand, within the abdomen, the drug unleash ought to be suppressed by a pH scale sensing perform (acid resistance) within the dose kind, which might cut back variation in stomachal continuance.24 Enteric coated time-release press coated (ETP) tablets, square measure composed of 3 elements, a drug containing core pill (rapid unleash function), the press coated swellable hydrophobic chemical compound layer (Hydroxy propyl group polysaccharide layer (HPC), time unleash function) Associate in Nursingd an enteric coating layer (acid resistance function).23,28 The pill doesn't unleash the drug within the abdomen because of the acid resistance of the outer enteric coating layer. when stomachal removal, the enteric coating layer speedily dissolves and also the viscus fluid begins to slowly erode the press coated chemical compound (HPC) layer. once the erosion front reaches the core pill, fast drug unleash happens since the erosion method takes an extended time as there's no drug unleash amount (lag phase) when stomachal removal. The period of lag section is controlled either by the burden or composition of the chemical compound (HPC) layer. (Fig. 1)

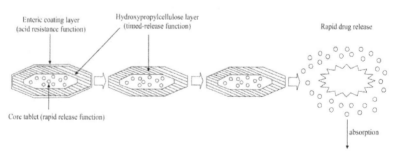

Fig 1: Design of enteric coated timed-release press coated tablet (ETP Tablet)

c. Microbially Triggered Drug Delivery to Colon:

The microflora of the colon is within the vary of 1011 -1012 CFU/mL, consisting chiefly of anaerobic bacterium, e.g. Bacteroides, bifidobacteria, eubacteria, clostridia, enterococci, enteric bacteria and ruminococcus etc.25 This large microflora fulfills its energy wants by zymosis numerous styles of substrates that are left undigested within the bowel, e.g. di- and tri-saccharides, polysaccharides etc.29,30 For this fermentation, the microflora produces a huge variety of enzymes like glucoronidase, xylosidase, arabinosidase, galactosidase, nitroreductase, azareducatase, deaminase, and carbamide dehydroxylase.31 attributable to the presence of the perishable enzymes solely within the colon, the employment of perishable polymers for colon-specific drug delivery appears to be a additional site-specific approach as compared to different approaches.5 These polymers defend the drug from the environments of abdomen and tiny gut, and area unit able to deliver the drug to the colon. On reaching the colon, they endure assimilation by micro-organism, or degradation by catalyst or break down of the compound back bone resulting in aensuant reduction in their mass and thereby loss of mechanical strength.32-36 they're then unable to carry the drug entity from now on.37

i) Prodrug Approach for Drug Delivery to Colon:

Prodrug is a pharmacologically inactive derivative of a parent drug molecule that requires spontaneous or enzymatic transformation in vivo to release the active drug. For colonic delivery, the prodrug is designed to undergo minimal hydrolysis in the upper tracts of GIT, and undergo enzymatic hydrolysis in the colon there by releasing the active drug moiety from the drug carrier. Metabolism of azo compounds by intestinal bacteria is one of the most extensively studied bacterial metabolic process.38 A number of other linkages susceptible to bacterial hydrolysis specially in the colon have been prepared where the drug is attached to hydrophobic moieties like amino acids, glucoronic acids, glucose, glactose, cellulose etc. Limitations of the prodrug approach is that it is not a very versatile approach as its formulation depends upon the functional group available on the drug moiety for chemical linkage. Furthermore, prodrugs are new chemical entities, and need a lot of evaluation before being used as carriers.39 A number of prodrugs have been outlined in Table 3.

9

Table 3: Prodrugs evaluated for colon specific drug delivery with there in vitro/in vivo performance

Carrier	Drug investigated	Linkage hydrolyzed	In vitro/in vivo model used	Performance of the Prodrug/conjugates
Azo conjugates Suphapyridine (SP) 5-ASA	5-ASA 5-ASA	Azo linkage Azo linkage	Human Human	Site specific with a lot of side effects40 associated with SP Delivers 2 molecules of 5-ASA as compared to suphasalazine41
Amino acid conjugates glycine	Salicylic acid	Amide linkage	Rabbit	Absorbed from upper GIT, though metabolized by microflora of large intestine42
Tyrosine/methionine	Salicylic acid	Amide linkage	Rabbit	Absorbed from upper GIT, though metabolized by microflora of large intestine43
L – Alanin/D-Alanine	Salicylic acid	Amid linkage	In vitro	Salicylic acid-l-alanine was hydrolysed to salicylic acid by intestinal microorganism but salicylic acid-D-alanine showed negligible hydrolysis thereby showing enantiospecific hydrolysis44
Glycine	5-ASA	Amid linkage	In vitro	Prodrug was stable in upper GIT and was hydrolysed by cecal content to release 5-ASA45
Saccharide carriers	Dexamethasone/prednisolone	Glycosidic linkage	Rat	Dexamethasone prodrug was site specific and 60% of oral dose reached the cecum. Only

Carrier	Drug investigated	Linkage hydrolyzed	In vitro/in vivo model used	Performance of the Prodrug/conjugates
				15% of prednisolone prodrug reached the cecum17
Giucose/galactose/ cellobioside	Dexamethasone; prednisolone hydrocortisone, fludrocortisone	Glycosidic linkage	In vitro	Less hydrolysis of the prodrug was seen in contents of stomach and proximal small intestine (PSI).hydrolysis increased in contents of distal small intestine (DSI) and was maximum in cecal content homogenates. galactosides hydrolyzed faster than glucosides which hydrolyzed faster than the corresponding cellobioside38
Glucuronide conjugates glucuronic acid	Naloxone/nalmefene	Glucuronide linkage	Rat	When given to morphine dependent rats, these reversed the GIT side effects caused by morphine without causing CNS withdrawal symptom because of activation in large intestine followed by a resultant diarrheas which excreted the prodrug 7 drug46
	Budesonide	Glucuronide linkage	Rat	Was found to be superior than budesonide itself for treatment of colitis47

(ii) Azo-Polymeric Prodrugs

Newer approaches are aimed at the use of polymers as drug carriers for drug delivery to the colon. Both synthetic as well as naturally occurring polymers have been used for this purpose. Sub synthetic polymers have been used to form polymeric prodrug with azo linkage between the polymer and drug moiety.48 These have been evaluated for CDDS. Various azo polymers have also been evaluated as coating materials over drug cores. These have been found to be similarly susceptible to cleavage by the azoreducatase in the large bowel. Coating of peptide capsules with polymers cross linked with azoaromatic group have been found to protect the drug from digestion in the stomach and small intestine. In the colon, the azo bonds are reduced, and the drug is released.28 A number of azo-polymeric prodrugs are outlined in Table 4.

Table 4: Some azo polymer-based drug delivery systems evaluated for colon-specific drug delivery with summary of results obtained

Azo polymer	Dosage from prepared	Drug investigated	In-vitro/in-vivo model used	Summary of the results obtained
Copolymers of styrene with 2-hydroxyethyl mrthacrylate	Coating over capsules	Vasopressin insulin	Rats dogs	These capsules showed biological respones characteristics of these peptide hormones in dog though it varied quantitatively49ˉ51
Hydrogels prepared by copolymerization of 2-hydroxyethyl methacrylate with 4-methacryloyloxy) azobenzene	Hydrogen	5-fluorouracil	In vitro	Drug release was faster and greater in human fecal media compared to simulated gastric and intestinal fluids52

12

Azo polymer	Dosage from prepared	Drug investigated	In-vitro/in-vivo model used	Summary of the results obtained
Segmented polynurethanes	Coating over pellets	Budesonide	Rat	These azopolymer-coated pellets were useful for colon-specific delivery of budesonide to bring healing in induced colites[53]
Aromatic azo bond containing urethane analogues	Degradable films	5-ASA	In vitro degradation of films in presence of lactobacillus	These films were degraded by azoreductase. The permeability of 5-ASA from lactobacillus treated films was significantly higher than that of control[54]

Open in a separate window

iii) Polysaccharide Based Delivery Systems

The use of naturally occurring polysaccharides is attracting a lot of attention for drug targeting the colon since these polymers of monosaccharides are found in abundance, have wide availability are inexpensive and are available in a vareity of a structures with varied properties. They can be easily modified chemically, biochemically, and are highly stable, safe, nontoxic, hydrophilic and gel forming and in addition, are biodegradable. These include naturally occurring polysaccharides obtained from plant (guar gum, inulin), animal (chitosan, chondrotin sulphate), algal (alginates) or microbial (dextran) origin. The polysaccrides can be broken down by the colonic microflora to simple saccharides.[21] Therefore, they fall into the category of "generally regarded as safe" (GRAS). A number of polysaccharide-based delivery systems have been outlined in Table 5.

Table 5: Polysaccrides investigated for colon specific drug delivery with their dosages forms and summary of results obtained

Polysaccharide investigated	Drug moiety used	Dosage form prepared	In vitro/ In vivo model used	Performance of the system
Chitosan	5-(6) carboxy fluorescein (CF)	Enteric-coated chitosan capsules	In-vitro	Little release of CF in upper GIT conditions and 100% drug release in 33% cecal contents within 4 h of dissolution55
Derivatives Chitson succinate Chitosan phthalate.	Sodium diclofenace	As matrices	In vitro	Reduced drug release was seen in acidic conditions and improved dissolutions under basic conditions56
Pectin (used as calcium salt)	Idomethacin	Matrices	In vitro	In the presence of rat cecal content drug release was 60.8±15.7% as compared to 4.9±1.1% in control57
Amidated pectin	Paracetamol	Matrix tablets	In vitro	These matrices were not suitable for drug delivery colon58
Amidated pectin / calcium pectinate	Ropivacaine	matrix tablet with ethyl cellulose as drug	In vitro	Amidated pectin were more susceptible to pectinolytic enzymes as compare to calcium pectinate. Addition of ethyle cellulose increased

14

Polysaccharide investigated	Drug moiety used	Dosage form prepared	In vitro/ In vivo model used	Performance of the system
		matrix additive		the tablets strength and dissolution rate coating this formulation with Eudragit L100 reduced drug release in upper GIT conditions without effecting enzyme degradability[59]
Chondroitin sulphate, Cross linked chondroitin Alginates As calcium salt	Indomethacin 5-ASA	Matrix tablet Double coated swellable beads	In vitro In vitro	Drug release increases in presence of rat cecal content. Also it was observed that as crosslinking increased, drug release decreased[60] In basic media enteric coating dissolves and beads swell to exceed the strength of aquacoat film, which then burst releasing the drug[61]

Open in a separate window

2. Newly Developed Approaches for CDDS

a. Pressure Controlled Drug-Delivery Systems

As a results of body process, higher pressures area unit encountered within the colon than within the intestine. Takaya et al. developed pressure controlled colon-delivery capsules ready victimization ethylcellulose, that is insoluble in water.[62] In such systems, drug unleash happens following the disintegration of a water-insoluble compound capsule due to pressure within the lumen of the colon. The thickness of the ethylcellulose membrane is that the most significant issue for the disintegration of- the formulation.63,64 The system additionally looked as if it would rely upon capsule size and density. due to resorption of water from the colon, the consistence of purple heart content is higher within the colon than within the intestine. it's thus been terminated that drug dissolution within the colon might gift a drag in relevance colon-specific oral drug delivery systems. In pressure controlled ethylcellulose single unit capsules the drug is during a liquid.65 Lag times of 3 to 5 hours in relevance drug absorption were noted once pressure-controlled capsules were administered to humans.

b. Novel Colon Targeted Delivery System (CODESTM)

CODESTM is an unique CDDS technology that was designed to avoid the inherent problems associated with pH or time dependent systems.66'67 CODESTM is a combined approach of pH dependent and microbially triggered CDDS. It has been developed by utilizing a unique mechanism involving lactulose, which acts as a trigger for site specific drug release in the colon, (Fig. 2). The system consists of a traditional tablet core containing lactulose, which is over coated with and acid soluble material, Eudragit E, and then subsequently overcoated with an enteric material, Eudragit L. The premise of the technology is that the enteric coating protects the tablet while it is located in the stomach and then dissolves quickly following gastric emptying. The acid soluble material coating then protects the preparation as it passes through the alkaline pH of the small intestine.68 Once the tablet arrives in the colon, the bacteria enzymetically degrade the polysaccharide (lactulose) into organic acid. This lowers the pH surrounding the system sufficient to effect the dissolution of the acid soluble coating and subsequent drug release.69

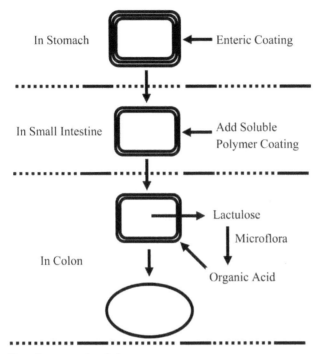

In Stomach — Enteric Coating

In Small Intestine — Add Soluble Polymer Coating

Lactulose

Microflora

In Colon

Organic Acid

Open in a separate window

Figure 2: Schematics of the conceptual design of CODES™

c. Osmotic Controlled Drug Delivery (ORDS-CT)

The OROS-CT (Alza corporation) can be used to target the drug locally to the colon for the treatment of disease or to achieve systemic absorption that is otherwise unattainable.[70] The OROS-CT system can be a single osmotic unit or may incorporate as many as 5-6 push-pull units, each 4 mm in diameter, encapsulated within a hard gelatin capsule, (Fig. 3).[71] Each bilayer push pull unit contains an osmotic push layer and a drug layer, both surrounded by a semipermeable membrane. An orifice is drilled through the membrane next to the drug layer. Immediately after the OROS-CT is swallowed, the gelatin capsule containing the push-pull units dissolves. Because of its drug-impermeable enteric coating, each push-pull unit is prevented from absorbing water in the acidic aqueous environment of the stomach, and hence no drug is delivered. As the unit enters the small intestine, the coating dissolves in this higher pH environment (pH >7), water enters the unit, causing the osmotic push compartment to swell, and concomitantly creates a flowable gel in the drug compartment. Swelling of the osmotic push compartment forces drug gel out of the orifice at a rate precisely controlled by the rate of water transport through the semipermeable membrane. For treating ulcerative colitis, each push pull unit is designed with a 3-4 h post gastric delay to prevent drug delivery in the small intestine. Drug release begins when the unit reaches the colon. OROS-CT units can maintain a constant release rate for up to 24 hours in the colon or can deliver drug over a period as short as four hours. Recently, new phase transited systems have come which promise to be a good tool for targeting drugs to the colon.72-75 Various in vitro / in vivo evaluation techniques have been developed and proposed to test the performance and stability of CDDS.

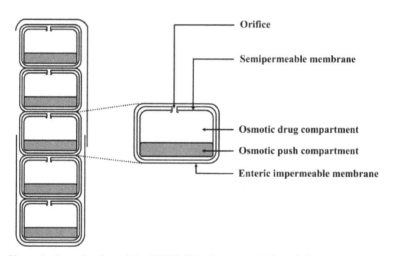

Figure 3: Cross-Section of the OROS-CT colon targeted drug delivery system

For in vitro evaluation, not any standardized evaluation technique is available for evaluation of CDDS because an ideal in vitro model should posses the in-vivo conditions of GIT such as pH, volume, stirring, bacteria, enzymes, enzyme activity, and other components of food. Generally, these conditions are influenced by the diet, physical stress, and these factors make it difficult to design a slandered in-vitro model. In vitro models used for CDDS are:

a) In vitro dissolution test

Dissolution of controlled-release formulations used for colon-specific drug delivery are usually complex, and the dissolution methods described in the USP cannot fully mimic in vivo conditions such as those relating to pH, bacterial environment and mixing forces.[69] Dissolution tests relating to CDDS may be carried out using the conventional basket method. Parallel dissolution studies in different buffers may be undertaken to characterize the behavior of formulations at different pH levels. Dissolution tests of a colon-specific formulation in various media simulating pH conditions and times likely to be encountered at various locations in the gastrointestinal tract have been studied.[76] The media chosen were, for example, pH 1.2 to simulate gastric fluid, pH 6.8 to simulate the jejunal region of the small intestine, and pH 7.2 to simulate the ileum segment. Enteric-coated capsules for CDDS have been investigated in a gradient dissolution study in three buffers. The capsules were tested for two hours at pH 1.2, then one hour at pH 6.8, and finally at pH 7.4.[77]

b) In vitro enzymatic tests

Incubate carrier drug system in fermenter containing suitable medium for bacteria (strectococcus faccium and B. Ovatus). The amount of drug released at different time intervals are determined. Drug release study is done in buffer medium containing enzymes (ezypectinase, dextranase), or rat or guinea pig or rabbit cecal contents. The amount of drug released in a particular time is determined, which is directly proportional to the rate of degradation of polymer carrier.

c) In vivo evaluation

A number of animals such as dogs, guinea pigs, rats, and pigs are used to evaluate the delivery of drug to colon because they resemble the anatomic and physiological conditions as well as the microflora of human GIT. While choosing a model for testing a CDDS, relative model for the colonic diseases should also be considered.

Guinea pigs are commonly used for experimental IBD model. The distribution of azoreductase and glucouronidase activity in the GIT of rat and rabbit is fairly comparable to that in the human.[78] For rapid evaluation of CDDS, a novel model has been proposed. In this model, the human fetal bowel is transplanted into a subcutaneous tullel on the back of thymic nude mice, which bascularizes within four weeks, matures, and becomes capable of developing of mucosal immune system from the host.

Drug Delivery Index (DDI) and Clinical Evaluation of Colon-Specific Drug Delivery Systems

DDI is a calculated pharmacokinetic parameter, following single or multiple dose of oral colonic prodrugs. DDI is the relative ratio of RCE (Relative colonic tissue exposure to the drug) to RSC (Relative amount of drug in blood i.e. that is relative systemic exposal to the drug). High drug DDI value indicates better colon drug delivery. Absorption of drugs from the colon is monitored by colonoscopy and intubation. Currently, gamma scintigraphy and high frequency capsules are the most preferred techniques employed to evaluate colon drug delivery systems.

2. LITERATURE REVIEW

1. Yachao Ren et al,.2017

The objective of this analysis was to style a brand new colon-targeted drug delivery system supported chitosan. The properties of the films were studied to get helpful data regarding the potential applications of composite films. The composite films were employed in a bilayer system to research their feasibleness as coating materials. durability, swelling degree, solubility, biodegradation degree, Fourier rework Infrared spectrographic analysis (FTIR), Differential Scanning mensuration (DSC), Scanning microscope (SEM) investigations showed that the composite film was shaped once chitosan and gelatin were reacted put together. The results showed that a 6:4 mix magnitude relation was the optimum chitosan/gelatin mix magnitude relation. In vitro drug unleash results indicated that the Eudragit- and chitosan/gelatin-bilayer coating system prevented drug unleash in simulated viscus fluid (SIF) and simulated stomachal fluid (SGF). However, the drug unleash from a bilayer-coated pill in SCF enlarged over time, and also the drug was nearly fully discharged when 24h. Overall, colon-targeted drug delivery was achieved by employing a chitosan/gelatin advanced film and a multilayer coating system.

2. Akhil Gupta et al,. 2017

Day by day there square measure new developments in field of colon specific drug delivery system. Colonic drug delivery has gained enlarged importance not only for the delivery of the medicine for the treatment of native unwellnesss related to the colon like Crohn's disease, inflammatory bowel disease, etc. however conjointly for the general delivery of proteins, therapeutic peptides, anti-asthmatic medicine, medication medicine and anti-diabetic agents. New systems and technologies are developed for colon targeting and to beat permeable method's limitations. Colon targeting holds an excellent potential and still would like a lot of innovative work. This critique discusses, in brief, introduction of colon, issue effecting colonic transition, colonic diseases and also the novel and rising technologies for colon targeting.

3. Venkateswara Reddy et.al.,2015

Colon targeted tablets were ready in 2 steps. at the start core tablets were ready then the tablets were coated by victimisation completely different pH dependent polymers. ethyl radical polysaccharide, Eudragit L100 and S100 were used as enteric coating polymers. The precompression mix of all formulations was subjected to numerous flow property tests and every one the formulations were passed the tests. The tablets were coated by victimisation polymers and also the coated tablets were subjected to numerous analysis techniques. The tablets were passed all the tests. Among all the formulations F3 formulation was found to be optimized because it was dim-witted the drug unleash up to twelve hours and showed most of 98.69% drug unleash. It followed zero order dynamics mechanism.

4. K. Satyanarayana Reddy et.al.,2015

Albendazole matrix tablets containing varied proportions of single blends of 3 pH sensitive polymers; Eudragit S100, radical radical methyl group polysaccharide Phthalate horsepower fifty five (HPMC Phthalate HP55), ethyl radical polysaccharide (Etcell), with completely different threshold pH 7.0, 6.8, 7.2 severally were ready by wet granulation technique involving drug compound magnitude relation studies in 1:1, 1:1.5, 1:2, 1:2.5 ratios. In vitro unleash profiles of Albendazole was consecutive determined in simulated stomachal fluid (SGF), simulated viscous fluid (SIF) pH 6.8 and simulated colonic fluid (SCF) pH7.2. The in vitro drug unleash from matrix tablets containing HPMC Phthalate HP55 and European Economic Community polymers showed unleash of 20-47% of Albendazole in Norse deity, followed by a burst unleash in SCF. However, matrix tablets containing compound blends Eudragit S100 showed that no considerable drug unleash occurred in Norse deity (0-20%). Among them, the formulations with drug compound ratios 1:2 and 1:2.5 showed a nominal unleash of drug in Norse deity one.3% and 0.27%. The formulation with drug compound magnitude relation 1:2 was elect as optimized formulation as a result of it showed a maximize unleash in proximal colon i.e. initial 2hrs in SCF and also the formulation with drug compound magnitude relation 1:2.5 showed associate degree extended unleash up to 3hrs in SCF successively missing the discharge within the target web site i.e. proximal colon.

5.   B. Manasa et.al. 2013

Prepared Matrix tablets by direct compression methodology. In-vitro studies disclosed that tablets developed with the natural polymers have controlled the drug unleash in abdomen and little gut atmosphere and discharged most quantity of the drug in colonic atmosphere. Results showed that tablets with higher binding concentration showed minimum drug unleash. Combination of polymers shows larger retarding of drug unleash. The soundness studies were distributed per the ICH pointers that indicates the chosen formulation (F10 & F12) were stable.

6.   Pranjal Kumar Singh et.al.,2012

Developed colon targeted film coated tablets of Motrin victimisation HPMC K4M, Eudragit L100, and ethyl radical polysaccharide as carriers. All the formulations (F1 to F6) were evaluated for the chemistry parameters and were subjected to in vitro drug unleash studies. the quantity of Motrin discharged from tablets at completely different time intervals was calculable by actinic ray photometer. The formulation F6 discharged 98.34 you look after Motrin. The results of the study showed that formulation F6 is presumably to produce targeting of Motrin for native action within the colon as a result of its nominal unleash of the drug within the initial five hrs.

7.   Mayur M Patel et al,. 2011

Oral colon-targeted drug delivery systems have gained monumental attention among researchers within the last 20 years. The importance of this site-specific drug delivery system are often measured by its utility for delivering a range of therapeutic agents, each for the treatment of native diseases or for general therapies. With the arrival of newer innovations, an oversized variety of breakthrough technologies have emerged for targeting a drug molecule to the colon. Researchers have tried varied approaches within the development of those formulation technologies, like pH-dependent, time-dependent and microflora-activated systems. Recently, variety of approaches are projected that utilize a unique construct of di-dependent drug delivery systems, that is, the systems during which the drug unleash is controlled by 2 factors: pH and time, and pH and microflora of the colon. This Editorial article isn't meant to supply a comprehensive review on drug delivery, however shall familiarise the readers with the formulation technologies that are developed for attaining colon-specific drug delivery.

8.   genus Rana Mazumder, et al., 2010

Have studied formulation and in vitro analysis of natural polymers based mostly microspheres for colonic drug delivery. The ready MTZ microspheres by ionotropic gelation technique were characterised by defence potency, particle size, micromaritic properties, in vitro unleash behavior, scanning microscopy, fourier transforms infrared spectrographic analysis.

9.   S. Lakshmana Prabu, et al., 2009

It was prompt the formulation and analysis of oral sustained unleash of calcium-channel blocker complex victimisation rosin as matrix forming material. Rosin could be a rosin used as a hydrophobic matrix material for the controlled unleash, victimisation diltizem HCL. Matrix tablets were ready by direct compression methodology victimisation rosin as matrix forming material in numerous magnitude relation. The rosin is beneficial in developing sustained unleash matrix tablets, it prolongs the discharge of water soluble drug up to 24h.

10.   Ziyaur Rahman,et.al., 2006

Core microspheres of alginate with 5-fluorouracil were ready by changed emulsification methodology in liquid paraffin followed by cross linking with salt. These core microspheres were coated with Eudragit s-100 by solvent evaporation technique. Drug unleash was sustained for up to twenty hours in formulations with core microspheres to Eudragit coat magnitude relation of 1:7 and no amendment in size, form and drug content were determined.

11.   H.N. Shivakumar, et.al.,2006

It absolutely was prompt the planning and analysis of pH sensitive multiparticulate system for chronotherapeutic delivery of diltiazepam complex. A pH sensitive multiparticulate system meant to approximate the chronobiology of cardiopathy is recommended for colon targeting. Core pellets was coated with crystalline polysaccharide and any coating of pellets victimisation Eudragit S -100. In-vitro dissolution studies of the coated pellets were performed following pH progression methodology. The drug unleash from the coated pellets depends on the coat weights and pH of the dissolution media.

12.   Sunil K. Jain,et.al.., 2004

Have studied preparation and analysis of Albendazole Microspheres for Colonic Delivery. Microspheres of Eudragit RL has developed for delivery of albendazole into the colon. The effects of compound concentration, stirring rate, and concentration of surfactant on particle size and drug loading has prompt.

13.   Fatemeh Atyabi, et.al.2004,

Rassoul Dinarvand., have ready ethyl radical polysaccharide coated gelatin microspheres as a multiparticulate colonic delivery system for 5-aminosalicilic acid. By solvent evaporation methodology were ready gelatin microspheres containing 5-aminosalicylic acid and also the ready microspheres were then coated with ethyl radical polysaccharide employing a coacervation-phase separation technique. it absolutely was shown that this technique might give an acceptable drug unleash pattern for colonic delivery of active agents,

14.   Y.S.R. Krishnaiah, et.al., 2002

Have developed oral colon targeted drug delivery systems for antiprotozoal victimisation gum as a carrier. Matrix, multilayer and compression coated tablets of antiprotozoal containing varied proportions of gum were ready. The results of the study showed that coated antiprotozoal tablets with gum of antiprotozoal for native action within the colon was simpler.

3. AIM AND OBJECTIVE

✓ The aim of the present research work was to develop sustained release matrix formulation of Pinaverium targeted to colon by using various polymers and in-vitro drug release study.

✓ The objective of this study was to prepare Pinaverium as a colon targeted tablet. Pinaverium matrix tablets containing several retarding agents separately were used in order to extend the release of drug over the desired period of time.

4. SCHEME OF WORK:

PART-I:

1.   Extensive literature survey.

2.   Procurement of excipients.

3.   Procurement of drug

PART-II:

Preformulation studies and Preparation of colon targeted tablets.

PART-III:

Evaluation of batches of colon targeted tablets containing Pinaverium for the following parameters

PART-IV:

Conclusion

Drug name : PINAVERIUM

Category : Alimentary Tract and Metabolism, Autonomic Agents, Calcium Channel Blockers

Synonyms : Dicetel, Eldicet, pinaverium, pinaverium bromide.

CAS NO : 59995-65-2

Structure :

Iupac-name: 4-[(2-bromo-4,5-dimethoxyphenyl)methyl]-4-[2-(2-{6,6-dimethylbicyclo[3.1.1]heptan-2-yl}ethoxy)ethyl]morpholin-4-ium

Molecular formula : $C_{26}H_{41}BrNO_4$

Molecular weight : Average: 511.52, Monoisotopic: 510.221348 g/mol.

Solubility : Soluble in DMSO, and methanol.

Melting point : 152-158⁰C

Bioavailability : less than 1%

Half-life : approximately 1.5 hours

Dosage forms & Dose : tablets-50, 100mg.

Pharmacokinetic Properties:

Absorption : After oral administration, pinaverium is poorly absorbed (5-10%) followed by uptake by liver. Poor absorption is due to its highly polar quaternary ammonium group and high molecular weight, which limits extensive diffusion across all cell membranes and promotes its selectivity towards the gastrointestinal tracts. Peak plasma concentration is reached within one hour after administration and the absolute oral bioavailability is reported to be less than 1%.

Distribution : It is selectively distributed to the digestive tract due to poor absorption and marked hepatobiliary excretion, Pinaverium is highly bound to human plasma proteins with the ratio of 97%

Metabolism : Hepatic metabolism of pinaverium involves demethylation of one of the methoxy groups, hydroxylation of the norpinanyl ring and elimination of the benzyl group with subsequent opening of the morpholine ring.

Elimination : Pinaverium is predominantly eliminated into feces

Adverse Effects : Some minor GI-related adverse effects include epigastric pain and/or fullness, nausea, constipation, heartburn, distension, and diarrhoea. Other side effects are headache, dry mouth, drowsiness, vertigo and skin allergy. Oral LD50 in mice, rats and rabbits are 1531 mg/kg, 1145 mg/kg and 154 mg/kg, respectively [L873]. Pinaverium displays no teratogenic, mutagenic or carcinogenic potential.

Storage : store at -20^0C

5.2. ETHYL CELLULOSE:

EC is a derivative of cellulose in which some of the hydroxyl groups on the repeating anhydroglucose units are modified into ethyl ether groups, largely called as non-ionic ethyl ether of cellulose.

EC has extensively been used for microencapsulation due to its many versatile properties such as(4):

1. white to light tan odorless and tasteless powder or granular substance;

2. melting point range 240-255^{0}C;

3. specific density range 1.07-1.18 with 135-155^{0}C heat distortion point and 330-360^{0}C fire point;

4. water insoluble but soluble in many organic solvents such as alcohol, ether, ketone and ester;

5. biocompatible and compatible with many celluloses, resin and almost all plasticizers;

6. non-biodegradable, thus used in oral formulation only;

7. stable against light, heat, oxygen and wetness and chemicals;

8. non-toxic;

9. non-irritant;

10. tablet binder to impart plastic flow properties to particles;

11. ability to absorb pressure and hence protect the coating from fracture during compression. Its thin

5.3. Cross Carmellose Sodium

Croscarmellose sodium should be defined as a cross-linked polymer of carboxymethyl cellulose. There are many differences between the starch and cellulose polymer and the important includes Differences between the synthetic processes that is used to modify the polymer. Most notably, the DS of croscarmellose sodium is greater than that of sodium starch glycolate, and the process of cross linking is changed. The substitution is implemented by Williamsons

30

ether synthesis to give the sodium salt of carboxymethyl cellulose. A significant change from the chemistry of SSG is that certain of the carboxymethyl groups themselves are utilise to cross-link the cellulose chains, the procedure being accomplished by dehydration. Thus, the crosslinks are carboxyl ester links relatively than phosphate ester links as in Primo gel.

5.4. EUDRAGIT RLPO, Eudragit L 100

These polymers allow the active in your solid dosage form to perform during the passage of the human body. The flexibility to combine the different polymers enables you to achieve the desired drug release profile by releasing the drug at the right place and at the right time and, if necessary, over a desired period of time. Other important functions are protection from external influences (moisture) or taste/odor masking to increase patient compliance. The range of our product portfolio provides full flexibility for your targeted drug release profiles by offering best performance for enteric, protective or sustained-release properties. EUDRAGIT® polymers are copolymers derived from esters of acrylic and methacrylic acid, whose physicochemical properties are determined by functional groups (R). EUDRAGIT® polymers are available in a wide range of different physical forms (aqueous dispersion, organic solution granules and powders). A distinction is made between 1. Poly(meth)acrylates; soluble in digestive fluids by salt formation EUDRAGIT® L, S, FS and E polymers with acidic or alkaline groups enable pH-dependent release of the active ingredient. EUDRAGIT® L and S polymers are your preferred choice of coating polymers. They enable targeting specific areas of the intestine. Pharma Polymers offers a broad product portfolio of anionic EUDRAGIT® grades which dissolve at rising pH values. In addition, the different grades can be combined with each other, making it possible to adjust the dissolution pH, and thus to achieve the required GI targeting for the drug. Targeted drug release in the colon is required for local treatment of intestinal disorders such as Crohn's disease, ulcerative colitis or intestinal cancer. It is also required for drugs that are poorly soluble in the upper gastrointestinal tract. Moreover, the gastroresistance of the coating ensures that the oral dosage form is patient compliant. The preferred coating is EUDRAGIT® FS 30 D, which combines release in the colon with the following technical advantages:

31

• aqueous processing

• highly flexible coatings

• suitable for multiparticulate tablet preparation

5.6. MAGNESIUM STEARATE

Flow agents help ensure a consistent dose of product in each capsule. Magnesium stearate does this by preventing individual ingredients from sticking to each other and from sticking to the encapsulating machines. It allows manufacturers to create a consistently homogenous mix, so the amount of active ingredients is the same from capsule to capsule or tablet to tablet. In other words, the use of magnesium stearate and other flow agents helps ensure consistency and quality control. Magnesium stearate is a simple salt made of two common nutritional substances, the mineral magnesium and the saturated fat stearic acid. It is used as a "flow agent" in many nutritional supplements and pharmaceuticals. Magnesium stearate contains two molecules of stearic acid and one molecule of magnesium. The molecule is held together by ionic bonds — the definition of a salt — that break apart easily in acid, the condition found in the human stomach. Though the name may make it sound like a synthetic, space-age molecule, both magnesium and stearic acid are abundantly available in many foods in our diet.

5.7. MICRO CRYSTALLINE CELLULOSE

Powdered cellulose and microcrystalline cellulose come from □-cellulose (cellulose free of hemi-celluloses and lignin) pulp from fibrous plant materials; they differ in regard to their manufacturing processes. Powdered cellulose is obtained by □-cellulose purification and mechanical size reduction. Crystalline cellulose is obtained by controlled hydrolysis of □cellulose with mineral acid solutions (2 to 2.5N), followed by hydrocellulose purification by filtration and spray-drying of the aqueous portion

In compounded medicines, powdered cellulose and microcrystalline cellulose are used as an adsorbent, a suspending agent, a capsule diluent (5-30% and 20-90%, respectively). Powdered cellulose is also used as a thickening agent. The applications of the powdered cellulose and the microcrystalline cellulose in compounding pharmacies include the oral solid dosage form (capsules) as a bulking agent to increase the mass in formulations containing small amounts of the active ingredient. The powdered cellulose is a base material for powder dosage forms, a suspending agent for aqueous peroral delivery and an adsorbent and thickening agent for topic preparations. Moreover, the microcrystalline cellulose is a constituent of the vehicle used for oral suspension.

5.8. TALC

Talc is a mineral with the composition of $3Mg0.4Si02.H2o$, and referred to as hydrous magnesium silicate (1). The structure consists of MgO sheet sandwiched between two silica sheets. Each layer is electrically neutral, and the adjacent layers are held together by only weak van der Waals forces (1). The mineral composition of talc may vary depending on the geographical source of the deposit (1,2). Impurities in the form of calcium silicate and calcium carbonate makes the powder abrasive, while iron oxide or magnesium ferric silicate makes talc greyish in appearance (1,2). Very finely powdered talc is boiled in 2% hydrochloric acid and subsequently in weaker hydrochloric acid solution to remove iron and other soluble impurities. Finally the talc is thoroughly washed with water and dried at 100°c (2). (For the variety of cosmetics products in which talc is a major component

MATERIALS:

Table& 5.2: List of Materials Used

Name of the material	Source
Pinaverium	sravs LABS
Ethyl Cellulose	Signet Chemical Corporation, Mumbai, India.
Eudragit RLPO	Merck Pvt Ltd, Mumbai, India.
Eudragit L-100	Merck Pvt Ltd, Mumbai, India.
Cross carmellose sodium	Merck Pvt Ltd, Mumbai, India
Magnesium stearate	Merck Pvt Ltd, Mumbai, India
Micro crystalline cellulose	Merck Pvt Ltd, Mumbai, India
Talc	Merck Pvt Ltd, Mumbai, India

Table 5.3: List of Equipment's used:

Name of the Equipment	Manufacturer
Weighing Balance	Wensar
Tablet Compression Machine (Multistation)	Karnavati, India.
Hardness tester	Monsanto, India.
Vernier calipers	Mitutoyo, Japan.
Roche Friabilator	Labindia, Mumbai, India
DissolutionApparatus	Labindia, Mumbai, India
UV-Visible Spectrophotometer	Labindia, Mumbai, India
pH meter	Labindia, Mumbai, India
FT-IR Spectrophotometer	Per kin Elmer, United States of America.

6. METHODOLOGY

Drug Polymer Compatibility Studies:-

Ø Drug polymer compatibility studies were carried out using FTIR.

Ø The study was carried out on individual pure drug and its physical mixture with the selected polymers under study.

UV Spectrum Analysis of Pinaverium:

The solution was scanned in the range of 200 to 400 nm to fix the maximum wave length and UV spectrum was obtained.

Reagents:

1) Standard Stocks – 1mg/ml in 0.1N HCl and 6.8 pH phosphate buffer.

2) Working Stocks – 100 ìg/ml in 0.1N HCl and 100 ìg/ml in 6.8 Ph phosphate buffer.

3) 0.1N HCl and 6.8 pH phosphate buffer.

From the working stock solutions, different aliquots of 0.5, 1, 1.5, 2.0 and 2.5 ml was taken in series of 10 ml volumetric flasks and volume was made up with 0.1N HCl and 6.8 pH phosphate buffers. The absorbance was obtained spectrophotometrically at 230 nm for 0.1N HCl and at 312 nm for 6.8 pH phosphate buffers respectively and calibration curves were constructed.

Formulation of core tablet:

The core tablets are formulated by using 50 mg of drug molecule, sodium starch glycollate as super disintegrate, Micro crystalline cellulose as diluent, talc and magnesium stearate as Glidant and Lubricant respectively. The composition of core tablet was given in below table.

Ingredient Name	Quantity (mg)
Pinaverium	50
Cross carmellose sodium	25
Talc	5
Magnesium stearate	5
MCC pH102	QS
Total weight	100

6.3. Composition of core tablet:

Total weight of core tablet was fixed as 100 mg. The tablets are prepared by using 9mm flat punch. Then the prepared core tablets are subjected to compression coating by using various compositions of polymers.

Formulation of compression coated tablets:

Table 6.4.Composition of coating layer:

Ingredient name	F1	F2	F3	F4	F5	F6	F7	F8	F9
Ethyl cellulose (mg)	50	100					50		50
Eudragit RLPO (mg)			50	10			50	50	
Eudragit L 100 (mg)					50	100		50	50
Magnesium stearate (mg)	6	6	6	6	6	6	6	6	6
Talc (mg)	6	6	6	6	6	6	6	6	6
MCC pH 102 (mg)	q.s	q.s	q.s	q.s	q.s	q.s	q.s	q.s	q.s
Total weight	200	200	200	200	200	200	200	200	200

Compression coating layer was divided into 2 equal parts i.e., 125mg of every amount .Half of the amount of powder mix was placed within the die cavity, core pill was placed specifically within the middle of die cavity then remaining amount of powder mix was placed over the core pill in order that the powder mix ought to cowl all facets|the edges|the perimeters} and high side of core pill uniformly. Then the pills square measure compressed by victimization 10mm flat surfaced punch victimization eight station tablet punching machine with the hardness of 4-4.5 kg/cm2.Then the ready compression coted tablets square measure evaluated for varied post compression parameters as per customary specifications.

EVALUATION OF COLON TARGETED TABLETS OF PINAVERIUM:

Micromeritic Properties:

Angle of Repose:

Determined by the funnel technique. The accurately ten g weighed powder taken in an exceedingly funnel. Height of the funnel was adjusted such the tip of the funnel simply touches the apex of the heap of powder. The powder was allowed to flow through funnel freely onto the surface. The diameter of the powder cone was measured and angle of repose was calculated exploitation the subsequent equation.

$$Tan\theta = h/r \text{------------- (1)}$$

Therefore, $\theta = Tan^{-1}h/r$

Where, θ = angle of repose, h = height of the cone r = radius of the cone base

Angle of repose in degrees	Type of flow
<25	Excellent
25-30	Good
30-40	Satisfactory
>40	Poor

Bulk Density:

Both loose bulk density (LBD) and tapped bulk density (TBD) were determined. A amount of ten g of powder from every formulation was introduced into a ten metric capacity unit mensuration cylinder. Initial volume was ascertained, the cylinder was allowed to faucet. The sound was continuing till no more amendment in volume was noted. Bulk density is calculated by victimization formula:

Weight of the powder

Bulk density (ρb) = Bulk volume of the powder

Weight of the powder

Tapped density (ρt) = tapped volume of the powder

Carr's Index:

The carr's index of the powder was determined by using formula:

Carr's index (%) = [(TBD – LBD) × 100]/TBD

Where, LBD = weight of the powder/volume of the packing

TBD = weight of the powder/tapped volume of the packing

Carr's index %	Type of flow
5-15	Excellent
12-18	Good
18-23	Satisfactory
23-35	Poor
35-38	Very poor
>40	Extremely poor

Evaluation of Physicochemical Parameters of Colon Targeted Tablets:

Tablet Thickness 5

Thickness was measured using screw gauze on 3 randomly selected samples.

Tablet Hardness 5

The hardness of tablet of each formulation was measured by pfizer hardness tester.

Friability 5

Roche friabilator was used for testing the friability. Twenty tablets were weighed accurately and placed in the tumbling apparatus that revolves at 25 rpm. After 4 min., the tablets were weighed and the percentage loss in tablet weight was determined.

$$\% \ loss = \frac{Initial\ wt.\ of\ tablets\ .\ Final\ wt.\ of\ tablets}{Initial\ wt.\ of\ tablets} * 100$$

Weight Variation 5

Twenty tablets were weighed individually and the average weight was determined. Then percentage deviation from the average weight was calculated. Deviation should not exceed the values given in table .

Average weight of tablet(mg)	Percentage deviation
80 mg or less	10
More than 80 mg but less than 250mg	7.5
250 mg or more	5

Uniformity of Drug Content 6

Five tablets were finely powdered; amount resembling fifty mg of pinaverium taken and dissolved with touch of vi.8 pH scale phosphate solution in to a a hundred millilitre of meter flask & created up to volume with vi.8 pH scale solution and mixed totally. one millilitre withdrawn & diluted to a hundred millilitre with vi.8 pH scale solution and measured the absorbance at the 312 nm employing a UV-visible photometer. The dimensionality equation obtained from activity curve was used for estimation of Pinaverium within the tablets formulations.

Dissolution Studies:

The release rate of pinaverium from tablets were determined exploitation USP dissolution testing equipment I (basket type). The take a look at was performed exploitation 900 metric capacity unit of 0.1 N HCl at 35 ± 0.5°C and a hundred rev for 1st two hrs. Then replaced with 6.8 pH scale phosphate buffer and continued for twenty-four hrs. Aliquot volume of ten metric capacity unit was withdrawn at regular intervals and replaced with recent buffer diluted. The samples were replaced with recent dissolution medium. once filtration, the number of drug unleash determined from the quality activity curve of pure drug.

7. RESULTS AND DISCUSSION:

7.1. Analytical Method:

Graphs of Pinaverium was taken in Simulated Gastric fluid (pH 1.2) and Simulated Intestinal Fluid (pH 6.8 and 7.4)

Table 7.1: Observations for graph of Pinaverium in 0.1N HCl (275 nm)

Conc [µg/l]	Abs
0	0
0.2	0.2107
0.4	0.4223
0.6	0.6402
0.8	0.8589
1	1.0601
1.2	1.2887

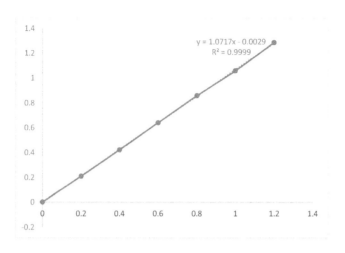

y = 1.0717x - 0.0029
R² = 0.9999

Figure 7.1: Standard graph of Pinaverium in 0.1N HCL

Figure 7.2: Standard graph of Pinaverium in 6.8 pH

Conc (mg/ml)	abs
0	0
0.2	0.144
0.4	0.271
0.6	0.398
0.8	0.519
1	0.643
1.2	0.771

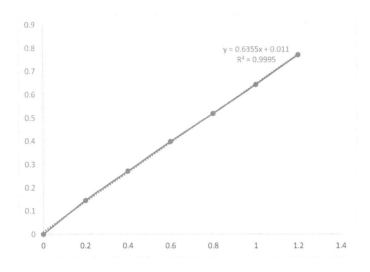

Figure 7.2: Standard graph of Pinaverium in 6.8 pH

7.2. Compatibility studies:

7.2.1 FT-IR spectrum of pure drug

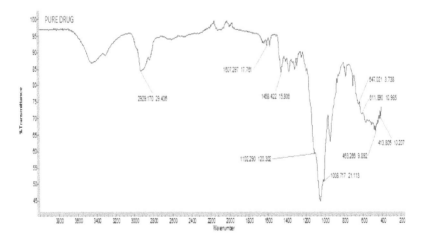

Figure 7.3. FT-IR Spectrum Of Pure Drug

7.2.2.FT-IR spectrum of optimized formulation

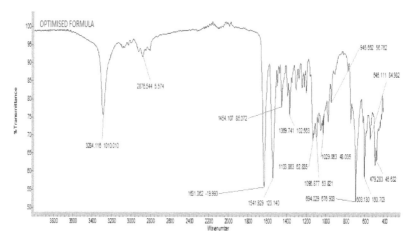

Figure :7.4: FT-IR spectrum of optimized formulation

The IR spectrum of pinaverium shows peaks at 3394 and 2929 cm⁻¹is due to H3CO Stretching, 3060 cm⁻¹ due to aromatic CH stretching, 2876 to 1507 cm⁻¹ due to CH stretching of CH3, H2 roups both symmetric and asymmetric and - 1468, 1369, 1102 cml- due to C=O Ring Stretching. Peak at 1649 cm⁻¹, 1610 cm⁻¹, 1442 cm⁻¹ and 687 cm⁻¹ are due to N-H bending , C=N bending, CH bending of CH3 and CH2 and C=O of CO-N-BR respectively. There was no noticeable change in the characteristic peaks of the pure drug in the optimized formulation hence considered compatible with the polymers used.

7.3. Pre-formulation parameters of core material:

Formulation Code	Angle of Repose	Bulk density (gm/ml)	Tapped density (gm/ml)	Carr's index (%)	Hausner's Ratio
F1	36.01	0.552±012	0.645±0.22	14.34±0.2	0.87±0.2
F2	31.8	0.574±0.34	0.664±0.26	13.16±0.3	0.82±0.4
F3	36.05	0.533±0.15	0.606±0.32	14.20±0.2	0.83±0.8
F4	34.22	0.531±0.16	0.613±0.24	13.60±0.5	0.86±0.3
F5	36.48	0.549±0.34	0.641±0.22	14.60±0.1	0.85±0.1

F6	33.40	0.564±0.24	0.666±0.21	15.62±0.2	0.85±0.2
F7	37.16	0.581±0.12	0.671±0.27	13.82±0.3	0.86±0.3
F8	35.24	0.567±0.21	0.654±0.19	13.24±0.4	0.84±0.7
F9	35.80	0.571±0.11	0.689±0.25	13.22±0.2	0.85±0.4

Table7.4: Pre-formulation parameters of Core blend

Pinaverium blend was subjected to various pre-formulation parameters. The apparent bulk density and tapped bulk density values ranged from 0.530 to 0.581 and 0.606 to 0.671 respectively. According to Tables 7.4, the results of angle of repose and compressibility index (%) ranged from 13.12 to 15.31. The results of angle of repose (<35) and compressibility index (<23) indicates fair to passable flow properties of the powder mixture. These results show that the powder mixture has good flow properties. The formulation blend was directly compressed to tablets and *in-vitro* drug release studies were performed.

7.5. Quality Control Parameters For compression coated tablets:

Tablet quality control tests such as weight variation, hardness, and friability, thickness, and drug release studies in different media were performed on the compression coated tablet. Total weight of tablet including core is 300 mg.

Formulation codes	Weight variation(mg)	Hardness (kg/cm2)	Friability (%loss)	Thickness (mm)	Drug content (%)
F1	312.5±0.22	4.5±0.2	0.52±0.24	4.8±0.03	99.24±0.21
F2	305.4±0.23	4.2±0.3	0.54±0.26	4.9±0.04	99.58±0.24
F3	298.6±0.14	4.4±0.2	0.51±0.24	4.9±0.01	99.48±0.22
F4	310.6±0.15	4.5±0.8	0.55±0.27	4.9±0.02	99.78±0.19
F5	309.4±0.22	4.4±0.1	0.56±0.21	4.7±0.05	99.57±0.18
F6	310.7±0.19	4.2±0.2	0.45±0.26	4.5±0.02	99.63±0.11
F7	302.3±0.15	4.1±0.6	0.51±0.26	4.4±0.06	98.41±0.24
F8	301.2±0.34	4.3±0.4	0.49±0.24	4.7±0.06	99.67±0.13
F9	298.3±0.21	4.5±0.2	0.55±0.22	4.6±0.01	99.24±0.22

7.4. Invitro quality control parameters for compression coated tablets:

All the parameters such as weight variation, friability, hardness, thickness and drug content were found to be within limits.

7.6 In-Vitro Drug Release Studies:

Time(hrs)	F1	F2	F3	F4	F5
1	6.19±0.3	0.73±0.1	0.34±0.5	3.39±0.7	1.11±0.5
2	23.16±0.1	2.46±0.3	0.54±0.1	19.88±0.5	2.49±0.7
3	38.49±0.4	11.46±0.5	1.26±0.3	36.45±0.1	18.19±0.5
4	56.34±0.5	28.19±0.4	2.22±0.5	49.59±0.3	31.19±0.1
5	68.44±0.7	45.79±0.8	3.05±0.4	59.01±0.1	42.46±0.3
6	80.16±0.8	62.87±0.5	18.41±0.1	69.85±0.3	56.78±0.7
7	88.17±0.5	76.19±0.1	30.05±0.3	79.46±0.7	66.19±0.4
8	98.14±0.1	85.16±0.3	48.69±0.7	86.19±0.4	79.46±0.7
9		92.78±0.1	55.32±0.3	99.14±0.5	91.46±0.7
10		97.73±0.4	72.34±0.1		96.10±0.5
11			87.56±0.4		
12			93.69±0.7		

Time(hrs)	F6	F7	F8	F9
1	1.44±0.1	8.06±0.5	2.65±0.3	1.32±0.1
2	12.30±0.7	20.46±0.3	10.23±0.1	1.74±0.4
3	24.44±0.3	34.46±0.1	19.19±0.4	3.67±0.7
4	36.61±0.1	48.41±0.3	31.57±0.5	9.57±0.5
5	47.30±0.4	68.76±0.1	43.08±0.3	19.48±0.7
6	55.68±0.5	76.73±0.4	58.74±0.1	31.87±0.3
7	67.53±0.8	94.23±0.5	65.13±0.3	52.47±0.1
8	78.72±0.7		78.45±0.1	62.46±0.4
9	83.35±0.5		85.67±0.4	73.44±0.5
10	90.67±0.1		98.42±0.7	83.44±0.1
11	96.12±0.3		98.12±0.5	92.47±0.3

| 12 | 98.45±0.8 | | | 96.44±0.4 |

Table 7.5: *In-vitro* **Drug Release profile for coated formulations (F1-F9)**

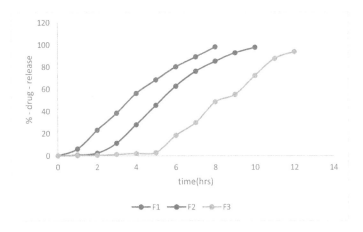

Fig 7.5 : Dissolution of formulations F1-F3

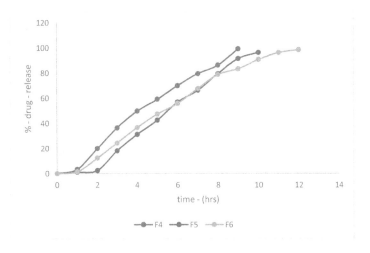

Fig 7.6 : Dissolution of formulations F4-F6

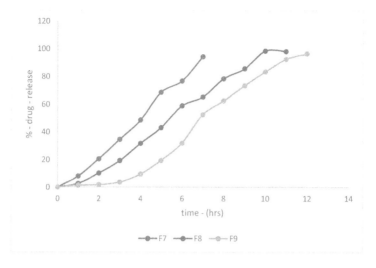

Fig 7.7 : Dissolution of formulations F7-F9

Application of Release Rate Kinetics to Dissolution Data:

Various models were tested for explaining the kinetics of drug release. To analyze the mechanism of the drug release rate kinetics of the dosage form, the obtained data were fitted into zero-order, first order, Higuchi, and Korsmeyer-Peppas release model.

Time (t)	root(t)	Cumulative (%) release q	log (t)	log(%) release	log(%) remain	release rate (cumulative % release / t)
0	0	0	0.000	0.000	2.000	0.000
1	1.000	1.44	0.000	0.158	1.994	1.440
2	1.414	12.3	0.301	1.090	1.943	6.150
3	1.732	24.44	0.477	1.388	1.878	8.147
4	2.000	36.61	0.602	1.564	1.802	9.153
5	2.236	47.3	0.699	1.675	1.722	9.460
6	2.449	55.68	0.778	1.746	1.647	9.280
7	2.646	67.53	0.845	1.829	1.511	9.647
8	2.828	78.72	0.903	1.896	1.328	9.840
9	3.000	83.34	0.954	1.921	1.222	9.260
10	3.162	90.67	1.000	1.957	0.970	9.067

48

11	3.317	96.12	1.041	1.983	0.589	8.738
12	3.464	98.45	1.079	1.993	0.190	8.204

Table 7.6: Release kinetics data for optimised formulation

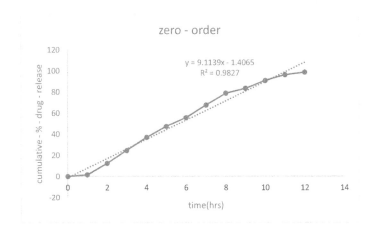

Fig 7.8 : Zero order release kinetics graph

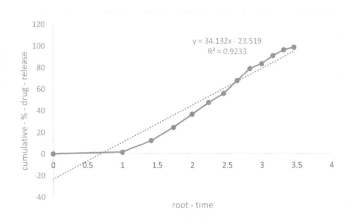

Fig 7.9: Higuchi release kinetics graph

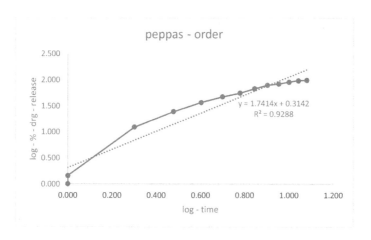

Fig 7.10: Kars mayer peppas graph

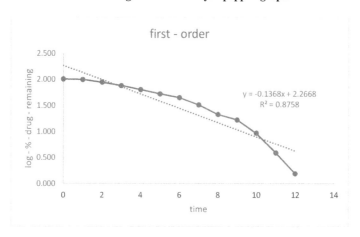

Fig 7.11: First order release kinetics graph

From the above graphs it was evident that the formulation F6 followed zero order drug release in kars mayer peppas mechanism.

8. CONCLUSION

• Sustained release matrix formulation of Pinaverium targeted to colon by using different polymers developed.

• To achieve pH-independent drug release of Pinaverium, hydrogen ion concentration modifying agents (buffering agents) were used.

• Colon targeted tablets were prepared in 2 steps. at first core tablets were prepared and so the tablets were coated by using different ph modifying polymers

• Ethyl polysaccharide, Eudragit L100 and S100 were used as enteric coating polymers.

• The pre-compression mix of all formulations was subjected to numerous flow property tests and every one the formulations were passed the tests.

• The tablets were coated by various polymers and also the coated tablets were subjected to numerous evaluation techniques.

• The tablets were passed all the tests.

• Among all the formulations F6 formulation was found to be optimized because its drug release is up to twelve hours and showed most of 98.45%dr.

• It followed zero order mechanism.

REFERENCES

1.   Philip AK, Dabas S, Pathak K. Optimized prodrug approach: a means for achieving enhanced anti-inflammatory potential in experimentally induced colitis. J Drug Target 2009. Apr;17(3):235-241 10.1080/10611860902718656

2.   Oluwatoyin AO, John TF. In vitro evaluation of khaya and albizia gums as compression coating for drug targeting to the colon. J Pharm Pharmacol 2005;57:63-168

3.   Akala EO, Elekwachi O, Chase V, Johnson H, Lazarre M, Scott K. Organic redox-initiated polymerization process for the fabrication of hydrogels for colon-specific drug delivery. Drug Dev Ind Pharm 2003. Apr;29(4):375-386 10.1081/DDC-120018373

4.   Chourasia MK, Jain SK. Pharmaceutical approaches to colon targeted drug delivery systems. J Pharm Pharm Sci 2003. Jan-Apr;6(1):33-66

5.   Basit A, Bloor J. Prespectives on colonic drug delivery, Business briefing. Pharmtech 2003; 185-190.

6.   Watts P, Illum L. Colonic drug delivery. Drug Dev Ind Pharm 1997;23:893-913 .10.3109/03639049709148695

7.   Wood E, Wilson CG, Hardy JG. The spreading of foam and solution enemas. Int J Pharm 1985;25:191-197 .10.1016/0378-5173(85)90092-4

8.   Chien YW. Oral drug delivery and delivery systems. In: Chien YW, editor. Novel drug delivery systems. New York: Marcel Dekker Inc; 1992; 139-196.

9.   Reddy SM, Sinha VR, Reddy DS. Novel oral colon-specific drug delivery systems for pharmacotherapy of peptide and nonpeptide drugs. Drugs Today (Barc) 1999. Jul;35(7):537-580

10.   Philip AK, Dubey RK, Pathak K. Optimizing delivery of flurbiprofen to the colon using a targeted prodrug approach. J Pharm Pharmacol 2008. May;60(5):607-613 10.1211/jpp.60.5.0006

11.   Kulkarni SK. Pharmacology of gastro-intestinal tract (GIT). In: Kulkarni SK. editor, Handbook of experimental pharmacology. New Delhi: Vallabh Prakashan; 1999; 148-150.

12.   McLeod AD, Friend DR, Tozer TN. Glucocorticoid-dextran conjugates as potential prodrugs for colon-specific delivery: hydrolysis in rat gastrointestinal tract contents. J Pharm Sci 1994. Sep;83(9):1284-1288 10.1002/jps.2600830919

13.   Vyas SP, Khar RK. Gastroretentive systems. In: Vyas SP, Khar RK, editors. Controlled drug delivery: concepts and advances. New Delhi: Vallabh Prakashan, 2005; 218-253.

14.   Antonin KH, Rak R, Bieck PR, Preiss R, Schenker U, Hastewell J, et al. The absorption of human calcitonin from the transverse colon of man. Int J Pharm 1996;130(1):33-39 .10.1016/0378-5173(95)04248-2

15.   Fara JW. Novel Drug Delivery and its Therapeutic Application. In: Presscot LF, Nimmo WS, editors. Colonic drug absorption and metabolism. Wiley: Chichester, 1989; 103-120.

16.   Mackay M, Tomlinson E. Colonic delivery of therapeutic peptides and proteins, In: Biek PR, editors. Colonic drug absorption and metabolism. New York: Marcel Dekker, 1993; 159-176.

17.   Friend DR, Chang GW. A colon-specific drug-delivery system based on drug glycosides and the glycosidases of colonic bacteria. J Med Chem 1984. Mar;27(3):261-266 10.1021/jm00369a005

18.   Rubinstein A. Approaches and opportunities in colon-specific drug delivery. Crit Rev Ther Drug Carrier Syst 1995;12(2-3):101-149

19.   Evans DF, Pye G, Bramley R, Clark AG, Dyson TJ, Hardcastle JD. Measurement of gastrointestinal pH profiles in normal ambulant human subjects. Gut 1988. Aug;29(8):1035-1041 10.1136/gut.29.8.1035

20.   Bussemer T, Otto I, Bodmeier R. Pulsatile drug-delivery systems. Crit Rev Ther Drug Carrier Syst 2001;18(5):433-458

21.   Ashord M, Fell JT, Attwood D, Sharma H, Woodhead P. An evaluation of pectin as a carrier for drug targeting to the colon. J Control Release 1993;26:213-220 .10.1016/0168-3659(93)90188-B

22.   Fukui E, Miyamura N, Kobayashi M. An in vitro investigation of the suitability of presscoated tablets with hydroxypropylmethylcellulose acetate succinate (HPMCAS) and hydrophobicn additives in the outer shell for colon targeting. J Control Rel 200; 70:97-107.

23.   Gazzaniga A, Iamartino P, Maffino G, Sangalli ME. Oral delayed release system for colonic specific drug delivery. Int J Pharm 1994;108:77-83 .10.1016/0378-5173(94)90418-9

24.   Fukui E, Miyamura N, Uemura K, Kobayashi M. Preparation of enteric coated timed-release press-coated tablets and evaluation of their function by in vitro and in

vivo tests for colon targeting. Int J Pharm 2000. Aug;204(1-2):7-15 10.1016/S0378-5173(00)00454-3

25.   Vassallo M, Camilleri M, Phillips SF, Brown ML, Chapman NJ, Thomforde GM. Transit through the proximal colon influences stool weight in the irritable bowel syndrome. Gastroenterology 1992. Jan;102(1):102-108

26.   von der Ohe MR, Camilleri M, Kvols LK, Thomforde GM. Motor dysfunction of the small bowel and colon in patients with the carcinoid syndrome and diarrhea. N Engl J Med 1993. Oct;329(15):1073-1078 10.1056/NEJM199310073291503

27.   Kinget R, Kalala W, Vervoort L, van den Mooter G. Colonic drug targeting. J Drug Target 1998;6(2):129-149 10.3109/10611869808997888

28.   Hita V, Singh R, Jain SK. Colonic targeting of metronidazole using azo aromatic polymers, development and characterization. Drug Deliv 1997;4:19-22 .10.3109/10717549709033183

29.   Rubinstein A. Microbially controlled drug delivery to the colon. Biopharm Drug Dispos 1990. Aug-Sep;11(6):465-475 10.1002/bdd.2510110602

30.   Cummings JH, Englyst HN. Fermentation in the human large intestine and the available substrates. Am J Clin Nutr 1987. May;45(5)(Suppl):1243-1255

31.   Scheline RR. Metabolism of foreign compounds by gastrointestinal microorganisms. Pharmacol Rev 1973. Dec;25(4):451-523

32.   Peters R, Kinget R. Film-forming polymers for colonic drug deliver: Synthesis and physical and chemical properties of methyl derivatives of Eudragit S. Int J Pharm 1993;94:125-134 .10.1016/0378-5173(93)90016-9

33.   Huang SI, Bansleben DA, Knox JR. Biodegradable polymers: Chymotrypsin degradation of low molecular weight poly (ester-urea) containing phenylalanine. J Appl Polym Sci 1979;23:429-437 .10.1002/app.1979.070230212

34.   Swift G. Biodegradable polymers in the environment: are they really biodegradable. Proc ACS Div Poly Mat Sci Eng 1992; 66:403-404.

35.   Ratner BD, Gladhill KW, Horbett TA. Analysis of in vitro enzymatic and oxidative degradation of polyurethanes. J Biomed Mater Res 1988. Jun;22(6):509-527 10.1002/jbm.820220607

36.   Hergenrother RW, Wabewr HD, Cooper SL. The effect of chain extenders and stabilizers on the in vivo stability of polyurethanes. J Appl Biomater 1992;3:17-22 .10.1002/jab.770030104

37.   Park K, Shalaby WS, Park H, eds. Biodegradation In: Biodegradable hydrogels for drug delivery, USA: Technomic publishing company, 1993; 13-34.

38.   Friend DR, Chang GW. Drug glycosides: potential prodrugs for colon-specific drug delivery. J Med Chem 1985. Jan;28(1):51-57 10.1021/jm00379a012

39.   Sinha VR, Kumria R. Microbially triggered drug delivery to the colon. Eur J Pharm Sci 2003. Jan;18(1):3-18 10.1016/S0928-0987(02)00221-X

40.   Khan AK, Piris J, Truelone SC. An experiment to determine the active therapeutic moiety of sulphasalazine. Lancet 1977;2:895-896

41.   Chan RP, Pope DJ, Gilbert AP, Sacra PJ, Baron JH, Lennard-Jones JE. Studies of two novel sulfasalazine analogs, ipsalazide and balsalazide. Dig Dis Sci 1983. Jul;28(7):609-615 10.1007/BF01299921

42.   Shibasaki J, Inoue Y, Kadosaki K, Sasaki H, Nakamura J. Hydrolysis of salicyluric acid in rabbit intestinal microorganisms. J Pharmacobiodyn 1985. Dec;8(12):989-995

43.   Nakamura J, Kido M, Nishida K, Sasaki H. Hydrolysis of salicylic acid tyrosine salicylic acid-methionine prodrug in rabbits. Int J Pharm 1992;87:59-66 .10.1016/0378-5173(92)90227-S

44.   Nakamura J, Tagami C, Nishida K, Sasaki H. Unequal hydrolysis of salicylic acid-D-alanine and salicylic acid-L-alanine conjugate in rabbit intestinal microorganisms. Chem Pharm Bull (Tokyo) 1992b Feb;40(2):547-549

45.   Jung YJ, Lee JS, Kim HH, Kim YM, Han SK. Synthesis and evaluation of 5-aminosalicyl-glycine as a potential colon-specific prodrug of 5-aminosalicylic acid. Arch Pharm Res 1998. Apr;21(2):174-178 10.1007/BF02974024

46.   Simpkins JW, Smulkowski M, Dixon R, Tuttle R. Evidence for the delivery of narcotic antagonists to the colon as their glucuronide conjugates. J Pharmacol Exp Ther 1988. Jan;244(1):195-205

47.   Cui N, Friend DR, Fedorak RN. A budesonide prodrug accelerates treatment of colitis in rats. Gut 1994. Oct;35(10):1439-1446 10.1136/gut.35.10.1439

48.   Van den Mooter G, Samyn C, Kinget R. In vivo evaluation of a colon-specific drug delivery system: an absorption study of theophylline from capsules coated with azo polymers in rats. Pharm Res 1995. Feb;12(2):244-247 10.1023/A:1016283027139

49.   Saffron M, Kumar GS, Savariora C, Burnham JC, Williams F, Neekers DC. A new approach to the oral administration of insulin and other peptide drugs. Sci 1986;233:1081-1084 .10.1126/science.3526553

50.   Saffran M, Bedra C, Kumar GS, Neckers DC. Vasopressin: a model for the study of effects of additives on the oral and rectal administration of peptide drugs. J Pharm Sci 1988. Jan;77(1):33-38 10.1002/jps.2600770107

51.   Saffran M, Field JB, Peña J, Jones RH, Okuda Y. Oral insulin in diabetic dogs. J Endocrinol 1991. Nov;131(2):267-278 10.1677/joe.0.1310267

52.   Shanta KL, Ravichandran P, Rao KP. Azopolymeric hydrogels for colon targeted drug delivery. Biomat 1995;16:1313-1318 .10.1016/0142-9612(95)91046-2

53.   Tozaki H, Fujita T, Komoike J, Kim SI, Terashima H, Muranishi S, et al. Colon-specific delivery of budesonide with azopolymer-coated pellets: therapeutic effects of budesonide with a novel dosage form against 2,4,6-trinitrobenzenesulphonic acid-induced   colitis   in   rats.   J   Pharm   Pharmacol   1999.   Mar;51(3):257-261 10.1211/0022357991772420

54.   Chavan MS, Sant VP, Nagarsenker MS. Azo-containing urethane analogues for colonic drug delivery: synthesis, characterization and in-vitro evaluation. J Pharm Pharmacol 2001. Jun;53(6):895-900 10.1211/0022357011776063

55.   Tozaki H, Komoike J, Tada C, Maruyama T, Terabe A, Suzuki T, et al. Chitosan capsules for colon-specific drug delivery: improvement of insulin absorption from the rat colon. J Pharm Sci 1997. Sep;86(9):1016-1021 10.1021/js970018g

56.   Aiedeh K, Taha MO. Synthesis of chitosan succinate and chitosan phthalate and their evaluation as suggested matrices in orally administered colon specific drug delivery   system.   Arch   Pharm   Res   1999;332:103-107   .10.1002/(SICI)1521-4184(19993)332:3<103::AID-ARDP103>3.0.CO;2-U

57.   Rubinstein A, Radai R, Ezra M, Pathak S, Rokem JS. In vitro evaluation of calcium pectinate: a potential colon-specific drug delivery carrier. Pharm Res 1993. Feb;10(2):258-263 10.1023/A:1018995029167

58.   Wakerly Z, Fell J, Attwood D, Parkins D. Studies on amidated pectins as potential carriers in colonic drug delivery. J Pharm Pharmacol 1997. Jun;49(6):622-625 10.1111/j.2042-7158.1997.tb06856.x

59.   Ahrabi SF, Madsen G, Dyrstad K, Sande SA, Graffner C. Development of pectin matrix tablets for colonic delivery of model drug ropivacaine. Eur J Pharm Sci 2000. Mar;10(1):43-52 10.1016/S0928-0987(99)00087-1

60.   Rubinstin A, Nakar D, Sintov A. Chondroitin sulphate: A potential biodegradable carrier for colon-specific drug delivery. Int J Pharm 1992;84:141-150 .10.1016/0378-5173(92)90054-6

61.   Shun YL, Ayres JW. Calcium alginate beads as core carriers of 5-aminosalicylic acid. Pharm Res 1992;9:714-790

62.   Takaya T, Niwa K, Muraoka M, Ogita I, Nagai N, Yano R, et al. Importance of dissolution process on systemic availability of drugs delivered by colon delivery system. J Control Release 1998. Jan;50(1-3):111-122 10.1016/S0168-3659(97)00123-5

63.   Muraoka M, Hu Z, Shimokawa T, Sekino S, Kurogoshi R, Kuboi Y, et al. Evaluation of intestinal pressure-controlled colon delivery capsule containing caffeine as a model drug in human volunteers. J Control Release 1998. Mar;52(1-2):119-129 10.

64.   Jeong Y, Ohno T, Hu Z, Yoshikawa Y, Shibata N, Nagata S, Takada K. Evaluation of an intestinal pressure-controlled colon delivery capsules prepared by a dipping method. J Control Rel 71(2):175-182.

65.   Hay DJ, Sharma H, Irving MH. Spread of steroid-containing foam after intrarectal administration. Br Med J 1979. Jun;1(6180):1751-1753 10.

66.   Watanabe S, Kawai H, Katsuma M, Fukui M. Colon specific drug release system. U. S. Patent, 1998, 09/183339.

67.   Takemura S, Watanabe S, Katsuma M, Fukui M. Human gastrointestinal treatment study of a novel colon delivery system (CODES) using scintography, Pro Int Sym Control Rel Bioact Mat 2000, 27.

68.   Katsuma M, Watanabe S, Takemura S, Sako K, Sawada T, Masuda Y, et al. Scintigraphic evaluation of a novel colon-targeted delivery system (CODES) in healthy volunteers. J Pharm Sci 2004. May;93(5):1287-1299 10.1002/jps.20063

69.   Yang L, Chu JS, Fix JA. Colon-specific drug delivery: new approaches and in vitro/in vivo evaluation. Int J Pharm 2002. Mar;235(1-2):1-15 10.1016/S0378-5173(02)00004-2

70.   Theeuwes F, Guittared G, Wong P. Delivery of drugs to colon by oral dosage forms. U. S. Patent, 4904474

71.   Swanson D, Barclay B, Wong P, Theeuwes F. Nifedipine gastrointestinal therapeutics system. Am J Med 1987;8(6):3 .10.1016/0002-9343(87)90629-2

72.   Philip AK, Pathak K. Osmotic flow through asymmetric membrane: a means for controlled delivery of drugs with varying solubility. AAPS PharmSciTech 2006;7(3):56 10.1208/pt070356

73.   Philip AK, Pathak K. In situ-formed asymmetric membrane capsule for osmotic release of poorly water-soluble drug. PDA J Pharm Sci Technol 2007. Jan-Feb;61(1):24-36

74.   Philip AK, Pathak K, Shakya P. Asymmetric membrane in membrane capsules: a means for achieving delayed and osmotic flow of cefadroxil. Eur J Pharm Biopharm 2008. Jun;69(2):658-666 10.1016/j.ejpb.2007.12.011

75.   Philip AK, Pathak K. Wet process-induced phase-transited drug delivery system: a means for achieving osmotic, controlled, and level A IVIVC for poorly water-soluble   drug.   Drug   Dev   Ind   Pharm   2008.   Jul;34(7):735-743 10.1080/03639040801911032

76.   Ahmed IS. Effect of simulated gastrointestinal conditions on drug release from pectin/ethylcellulose as film coating for drug delivery to the colon. Drug Dev Ind Pharm 2005. May;31(4-5):465-470 10.1080/03639040500214704

77.   Cole ET, Scott RA, Connor AL, Wilding IR, Petereit HU, Schminke C, et al. Enteric coated HPMC capsules designed to achieve intestinal targeting. Int J Pharm 2002. Jan;231(1):83-95 10.1016/S0378-5173(01)00871-7

78.   Mooter VG, Kinget R. Oral colon-specific drug delivery: A review. Drug Deliv 1995;2:881-931

79.   Yachao Ren, Lei Jiang, style and preparation of a unique colon-targeted pill of Cortef, Braz. J. Pharm. Sci. 2017;53(1):e15009.

80.   Akhil Gupta, Anuj Mittal, Alok Kumar Gupta, COLON TARGETED DRUG DELIVERY SYSTEMS —A REVIEW, Russian Journal of Biopharmaceuticals 3(4) · June 2011.

81.   Mayur M Patel (2011) up-to-date technologies in colon-targeted drug delivery systems, knowledgeable Opinion on Drug Delivery, 8:10, 1247-1258.

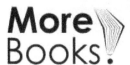

CPSIA information can be obtained
at www.ICGtesting.com
Printed in the USA
LVHW022303160523
747206LV00004B/214